The
MINDFUL
EATING
JOURNAL

The
MINDFUL
EATING
JOURNAL

PROMPTS *and* PRACTICES *to* RESTORE YOUR RELATIONSHIP *with* FOOD

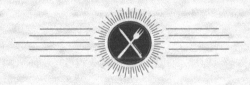

Alyssa Snow Callahan, MS, RDN

ROCKRIDGE
PRESS

Interior and Cover Designer: Karmen Lizzul
Art Producer: Sara Feintstein
Editor: Lia Ottaviano
Production Editor: Emily Sheehan
Author photo courtesy of © Les Schwartz.

ISBN: Print 978-1-64611-680-5
R0

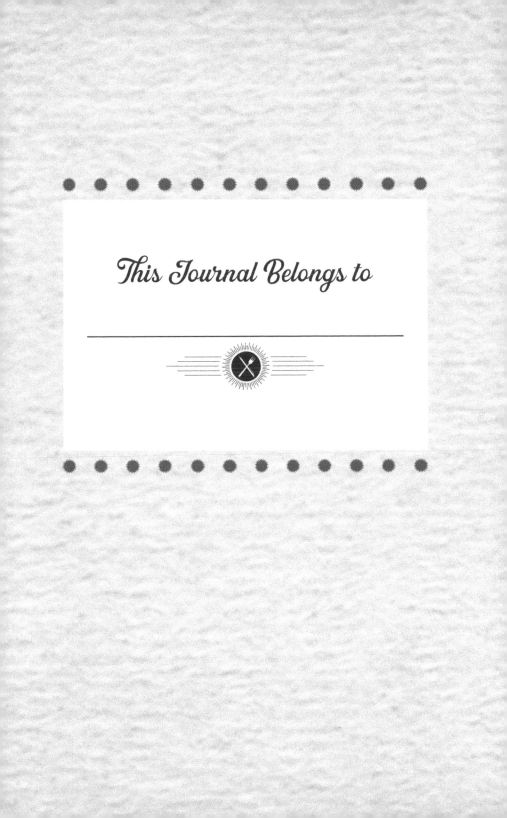

This Journal Belongs to

_____

To those in recovery from an eating disorder or disordered eating, those on the path to recovery, supportive loved ones, and those working in the recovery field, with all my loving kindness.

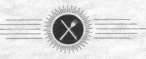

CONTENTS

Dear Reader,

Thank you for starting this journey to build a better relationship with food with me. I'm Alyssa, a registered dietitian nutritionist and certified intuitive eating counselor specializing in eating disorders, mindful eating, and body image. After struggling with an eating disorder, I spent years repairing my negative self-image and bridging the disconnect between my mind and my body. I know firsthand how difficult it can be to trust your body and love food again. That's why I am honored to join you on this journey and guide you in developing a daily practice of awareness, self-compassion, and gratitude around food and, ultimately, your body and yourself.

Food not only nourishes our bodies but also touches every part of our lives. Our choices around food reflect the social, cultural, financial, emotional, and spiritual parts of ourselves. This journal will lead you to reflect on current behaviors and choices around food and where your struggles are. More importantly, you will become aware of the thoughts and emotions that influence your relationship with food. Many of us develop a critical voice as a result of dieting or living in a culture that idolizes thinness and "health" extremes that don't actually align with how our bodies and brains function to keep us nourished. By identifying our food-related rules and beliefs, we can then decide whether these thoughts align with our values and benefit us or whether they are damaging to our self-worth and cause emotional distress. Learning to call out our inner critics as inaccurate and harmful is an important step in taking back our relationship with food, building trust with our bodies, and honoring our needs without judgment.

Although I specialize in working with clients with eating disorders, some of the work in this journal relating to listening to hunger and fullness cues may not be appropriate for those who are early in the eating disorder recovery process. I recommend discussing any work in this journal with your physician, therapist, and/or dietitian.

This journal isn't a substitute for medication or any medical or therapeutic treatment you can receive by working with a licensed professional. If the prompts in this book are meaningful to you, I suggest working with a dietitian and therapist who specialize in disordered eating to further the work you are starting with this journal. Working with a therapist or dietitian can help you process your struggles, address barriers, and obtain support along the way. There are many professionals who specialize in eating issues like I do, and we would absolutely love to help you. I've provided a few websites in the resources at the end of this journal to help you find a wonderful provider near you.

This journal is a journey in exploring your relationship with food, so try to use it regularly and give yourself time to enjoy the process. Many of the practices and meditations will be useful around mealtimes, so take extra time at meals and snacks to open your journal and reflect. Smell the aromas, feel accomplished with every entry, and be kind to yourself as you move at your own pace.

"Find the love you seek, by first finding the love within yourself. Learn to rest in that place within you that is your true home."

—SRI SRI RAVI SHANKAR

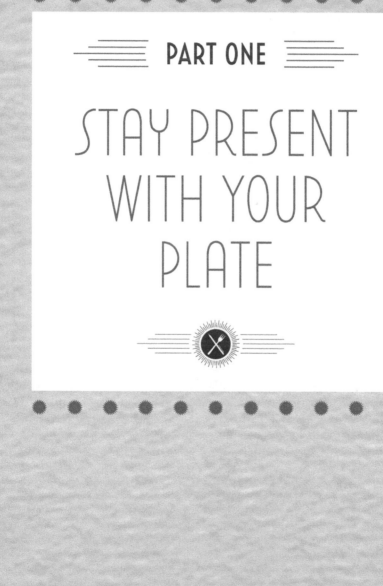

PART ONE

STAY PRESENT WITH YOUR PLATE

According to the principles of *Intuitive Eating*, developed by dietitians Evelyn Tribole and Elyse Resch, we are all born as mindful, intuitive eaters, listening to our bodies as a way to survive.[1] When infants are hungry, their discomfort causes them to cry so their caregivers know to feed them. Babies don't pass judgment on what they are eating or how much. They are present, listening to their bodies' signals, tasting their food, and bonding with their caregiver. When their needs are met, they are satisfied and can shift focus to another need. Put simply, this is mindful eating. Amazingly, you already know how to do this—you were born with this gift! Unfortunately, this wisdom is disrupted as we get older by messages from our families, friends, medical professionals, and, of course, our diet-loving, image-obsessed culture that tell us that our bodies are wrong and our inner knowledge can't be trusted. This couldn't be further from the truth. In fact, research finds that listening to our bodies' cues and dismantling these flawed food beliefs improves physical and mental health.[2,3,4] This section will guide you in finding your inner wisdom again and identifying steps you can take to stay connected with your needs.

"You must be completely awake
in the present to enjoy the tea.
Only in the awareness of the present,
can your hands feel the pleasant
warmth of the cup. Only in the present,
can you savor the aroma, taste the
sweetness, appreciate the delicacy.
If you are ruminating about the past,
or worrying about the future, you will
completely miss the experience
of enjoying the cup of tea.
You will look down at the cup,
and the tea will be gone."

—THICH NHAT HANH

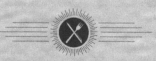

What are your goals for using this journal? How would you like your relationship with food to change by the time you complete the journal? Why do you want to make these changes? What would becoming a mindful eater mean to you?

_____

_____

_____

_____

_____

_____

_____

_____

_____

_____

_____

_____

_____

_____

_____

_____

_____

_____

_____

_____

Envision yourself as a mindful eater. What does it look like? What food are you eating? Where are you eating? Are you alone or with others? What looks different? What looks the same? How do you feel while you are eating?

_____

_____

_____

_____

_____

_____

_____

_____

_____

_____

_____

_____

_____

_____

_____

_____

_____

_____

_____

_____

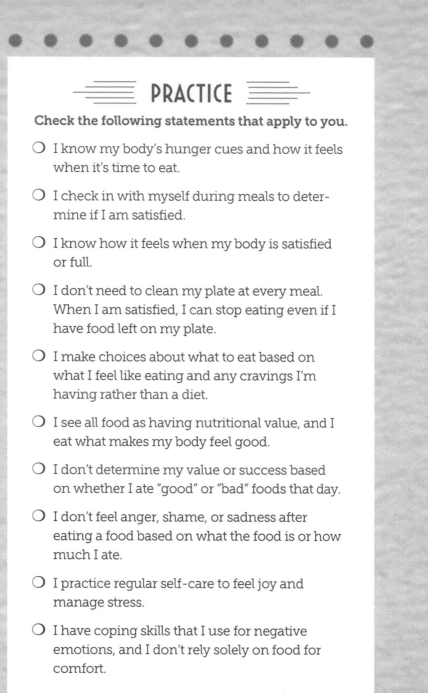

PRACTICE

Check the following statements that apply to you.

○ I know my body's hunger cues and how it feels when it's time to eat.

○ I check in with myself during meals to determine if I am satisfied.

○ I know how it feels when my body is satisfied or full.

○ I don't need to clean my plate at every meal. When I am satisfied, I can stop eating even if I have food left on my plate.

○ I make choices about what to eat based on what I feel like eating and any cravings I'm having rather than a diet.

○ I see all food as having nutritional value, and I eat what makes my body feel good.

○ I don't determine my value or success based on whether I ate "good" or "bad" foods that day.

○ I don't feel anger, shame, or sadness after eating a food based on what the food is or how much I ate.

○ I practice regular self-care to feel joy and manage stress.

○ I have coping skills that I use for negative emotions, and I don't rely solely on food for comfort.

Reflect on the statements that are not checked. Have you considered any of these goals in the past? What thoughts do you have as we start to incorporate these concepts into your eating patterns? Circle your top three goals from this list (even if you have others that aren't on this list).

_____

_____

_____

_____

_____

_____

_____

_____

_____

_____

_____

_____

_____

_____

_____

_____

_____

_____

_____

Think about you and food as having a back-and-forth relationship. What do you love about food? What positive role does this
relationship play in your life? Think about positive memories
and experiences relating to food.

_____

_____

_____

_____

_____

_____

_____

_____

_____

_____

_____

_____

_____

_____

_____

_____

_____

_____

_____

On the other side, how is your relationship with food toxic? How does food relate to your negative emotions (such as shame, sadness, anger, anxiety, or insecurity)?

_____

_____

_____

_____

_____

_____

_____

_____

_____

_____

_____

_____

_____

_____

_____

_____

_____

_____

_____

_____

Our values shape our view of the world, our relationships, and our behaviors. Our daily lives are structured around our values, such as spending quality time with loved ones, pursuing physical and mental health, giving back to those in need, and having a strong work ethic. How do your current thoughts and actions around food reflect your values? How might they contradict your values?

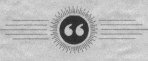

"Trust yourself. You know more than you think you do."

—BENJAMIN SPOCK

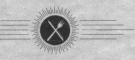

What does hunger feel like in your body? What sensations are present and where? (Start by noticing feelings in your stomach and your head.) Compare the sensations with different levels of hunger, such as feeling slightly hungry and ready for a snack, hungry enough for a meal, and overwhelmingly hungry or "starving."

_____

_____

_____

_____

_____

_____

_____

_____

_____

_____

_____

_____

_____

_____

_____

_____

_____

_____

Let's reflect on any judgment that might accompany feeling hungry. What do you normally do when you feel hungry? Do you always allow yourself to eat without judgment, even when it's not around a typical mealtime? What thoughts or emotions arise when you get hungry?

_____

_____

_____

_____

_____

_____

_____

_____

_____

_____

_____

_____

_____

_____

_____

_____

_____

_____

_____

Think of a situation when you were uncomfortably hungry. What do you think led to that experience? Did you have limited time, no access to food, or were you dealing with a negative emotion? What can you learn from this experience?

_____

_____

_____

_____

_____

_____

_____

_____

_____

_____

_____

_____

_____

_____

_____

_____

_____

_____

_____

_____

_____

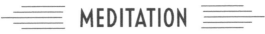 MEDITATION

Let's take a moment to check in with ourselves. Take a deep breath. Sit back in your seat, get comfortable, and feel the ground beneath your feet. Begin focusing on your breath, taking in fresh air and exhaling at a natural pace. Notice any physical sensations. Start with your head and scan your body down to your toes. If you feel any tension, send attention there and feel free to adjust your body to be more comfortable. Notice any thoughts that come to mind. Don't engage the thoughts; just observe them and return your focus to your breath. Notice your emotions. Try to visualize yourself releasing any negativity each time you exhale. Continue focusing on your breathing and any sensations you experience. Allow yourself to feel connected to your body.

Now let's consider fullness. What does fullness feel like in your body? What sensations are present and where? Compare the sensations with different levels of fullness, such as feeling slightly satisfied, full after a meal, and overwhelmingly full or "stuffed."

Are there any judgmental thoughts that accompany feeling full? What thoughts or emotions arise when you are full? Does it change based on how full you are? What do you think has influenced those thoughts about fullness?

_____

_____

_____

_____

_____

_____

_____

_____

_____

_____

_____

_____

_____

_____

_____

_____

_____

_____

_____

"There is a voice that doesn't use words. Listen."

—RUMI

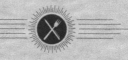

Think of a time when you were uncomfortably full. What led to this experience? Was it being too hungry before the meal, eating too quickly, finding comfort or joy in that food, or dealing with a negative emotion? What can you learn from this experience?

_____

_____

_____

_____

_____

_____

_____

_____

_____

_____

_____

_____

_____

_____

_____

_____

_____

_____

_____

_____

Consider the varying levels of hunger and fullness we've explored, from painfully hungry to painfully full and all the sensations in between. What sensations do you identify as feeling most often? Do you usually notice your feelings of subtle hunger and fullness? How can you stay connected with your hunger/fullness cues throughout the day?

_____

_____

_____

_____

_____

_____

_____

_____

_____

_____

_____

_____

_____

_____

_____

_____

_____

_____

MANTRA

Every meal and snack is an opportunity for learning more about our body's cues, our emotions, and how they affect one another. There are no mistakes or failures.

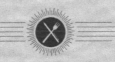

Think of your typical weekday. How do you typically decide when, where, and what to eat? Do you follow a typical eating schedule every day or do you play it by ear? What influences your choices?

_____

_____

_____

_____

_____

_____

_____

_____

_____

_____

_____

_____

_____

_____

_____

_____

_____

_____

_____

Now consider your typical weekend day. How do you typically decide when, where, and what to eat? Does it differ from your weekday strategy?

_____

_____

_____

_____

_____

_____

_____

_____

_____

_____

_____

_____

_____

_____

_____

_____

_____

_____

_____

_____

After considering your current decision-making strategies and schedules, how would you like your choices around meals and snacks to change to be more in tune with your body? What are simple steps you can start with?

_____

_____

_____

_____

_____

_____

_____

_____

_____

_____

_____

_____

_____

_____

_____

_____

_____

_____

_____

_____

"Who looks outside, dreams;
who looks inside, awakes."

—CARL GUSTAV JUNG

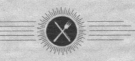

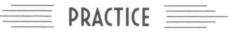

PRACTICE

Use the meditation earlier in this section to check in before you eat a meal. How hungry do you feel? Where do you feel it in your body? Are there any thoughts or emotions arising? Begin eating and take a break when you are finished with a third of your food. Put down your utensil and check in with your body's sensations, thoughts, and emotions again. Eat another third and check in. Based on your hunger and fullness, continue eating until your meal is finished or until you are satisfied or full. Check in again. If you are still hungry, get more food and eat until you are satisfied or full, making time to check in again if needed. When you're satisfied, check in again. How full do you feel? What sensations are present in your body? What emotions and thoughts are present?

_____

_____

_____

_____

_____

_____

_____

Reflect on your experience checking in throughout a meal. What did you learn? Compare how the meal went compared to meals when you haven't checked in.

_____

_____

_____

_____

_____

_____

_____

_____

_____

_____

_____

_____

_____

_____

_____

_____

_____

_____

_____

_____

_____

_____

_____

What can you do to give yourself time and support in regularly checking in with your hunger, fullness, and emotions before, during, and after every meal? What barriers can you anticipate and how will you address them?

_____

_____

_____

_____

_____

_____

_____

_____

_____

_____

_____

_____

_____

_____

_____

_____

_____

_____

_____

_____

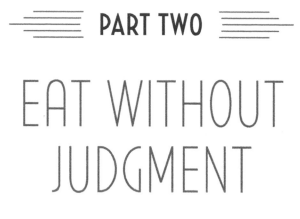

PART TWO

EAT WITHOUT JUDGMENT

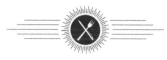

N ow that we have started connecting with our bodies to be intentional about our food-related choices and actions, we need to address our thoughts. This is when we start dismantling that critical voice that tells us to listen to external "diet" rules and not our own bodies' signals. This process is crucial, as dieting rules contradict how our brains function to keep us nourished. As humans, we require a variety of foods containing carbohydrates, protein, fat, vitamins, and minerals to meet all of our bodies' needs. Cutting out major food groups sets us up for craving the foods we are restricting because our brains tell us we need these foods for our bodies to function at their best. For example, we can't subsist on fruits and vegetables alone—our bodies require fats for making hormones and protecting our organs, proteins for repairing muscles and skin tissue, and carbohydrates to fuel our brains, among many other reasons. Often our body functions worsen due to nutritional deficiencies, leading us to give in to increasingly strong cravings. It is the deprivation of food, not the food itself, that causes us to overeat and have intense food cravings.[5,6] Yet we demonize food, criticize our bodies, and blame ourselves. We feel ashamed, thinking that we failed the diet, when in fact it was the other way around. These judgmental thoughts turn into negative beliefs and destructive talk about food and ourselves. Research has found dieting to be a risk factor for developing eating disorders or disordered eating habits in adolescence into adulthood, while eating intuitively is related to fewer eating disorder behaviors.[7,8] With mindfulness, all foods and choices are equal. Your awareness of your body and mind guides your choices so you can experience all foods with curiosity. This section will help you take a step back and reconsider your food rules and restructure your mind to eat without judgment.

"*For there is nothing either good or bad, but thinking makes it so.*"

—WILLIAM SHAKESPEARE, *HAMLET*

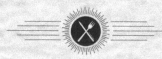

What was the first time you can remember thinking certain foods or food groups were "good" or "bad"? Where did these messages come from?

_____

_____

_____

_____

_____

_____

_____

_____

_____

_____

_____

_____

_____

_____

_____

_____

_____

_____

_____

_____

_____

Think about your childhood. What was your family's food culture like? Were there any rules about food or meals? Do you agree with them or continue to follow them now? Are there any rules that you no longer follow or wish not to follow anymore?

_____

_____

_____

_____

_____

_____

_____

_____

_____

_____

_____

_____

_____

_____

_____

_____

_____

_____

_____

_____

Now reflect on what is helpful and potentially damaging about your current food culture. How do people around you now (such as friends, family, and coworkers) talk about food? Does anyone eat mindfully, or do they follow strict diets? Are there any food rules imposed on you?

_____

_____

_____

_____

_____

_____

_____

_____

_____

_____

_____

_____

_____

_____

_____

_____

_____

_____

_____

PRACTICE

List your food-related rules, including "good" and "bad" foods. Identify where each belief comes from (e.g., culture, family, friends, past diets) and your current reason for believing or following it. Label each rule as helpful, hurtful, or unsure. Put a star next to each rule you're open to breaking.

_____

_____

_____

_____

_____

_____

_____

_____

_____

_____

_____

_____

_____

Have you had experience with dieting? What made you first feel like you needed to be "on a diet" or change your eating habits to alter your body? What diets have you tried? What have been the results of each diet? Were these results sustainable? Make a chart or timeline of changes in your diet and exercise routines and any effects on you, including your energy levels, physical strength, feeling connected to your body, and how you felt about yourself.

_____

_____

_____

_____

_____

_____

_____

_____

_____

_____

_____

_____

_____

_____

_____

_____

_____

Have you ever felt like you "failed" a diet? What caused you to end the diet? How did you feel after you stopped? What happened after you started eating "normally" again?

_____

_____

_____

_____

_____

_____

_____

_____

_____

_____

_____

_____

_____

_____

_____

_____

_____

_____

_____

_____

Have you ever considered that diets are actually failing you? Do you think the diets ultimately helped or harmed your relationship with food?

_____

_____

_____

_____

_____

_____

_____

_____

_____

_____

_____

_____

_____

_____

_____

_____

_____

_____

_____

_____

"The world as we have created it is a process of our thinking. It cannot be changed without changing our thinking."

—ALBERT EINSTEIN

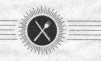

How did dieting serve you in the past? For instance, it may have provided hope, comfort, or structure. Explore how dieting may no longer be helpful in your life.

Think about when you have been on a diet that caused you to cut out a certain food group. How does avoiding a food group affect your mood, feelings, cravings, or behaviors?

_____

_____

_____

_____

_____

_____

_____

_____

_____

_____

_____

_____

_____

_____

_____

_____

_____

_____

_____

_____

MEDITATION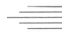

Diets feed into a perfectionist mindset. If only we could follow the rules perfectly and eat "perfectly," then we would feel our best and look "perfect." Unfortunately, this mentality only sets us up for feelings of failure and inadequacy. How would your life look if there were no "perfect" diet or body type that you have to strive for? Draw a picture or a word cloud (a cluster of meaningful words) of what a balanced life would mean to you. If you're stuck, start with drawing a balanced plate for one of your meals, and then draw another plate of ingredients for a balanced life.

Have you ever overeaten a food after a diet where you couldn't have that food? Have you ever overeaten a food leading up to a diet that prohibited that food? Reflect on how you felt in these situations.

_____

_____

_____

_____

_____

_____

_____

_____

_____

_____

_____

_____

_____

_____

_____

_____

_____

_____

_____

_____

_____

What foods do you tend to crave? Reflect on how these cravings may relate to favorite flavor profiles or textures, past diets, your food rules, or any feelings around those foods.

_____

_____

_____

_____

_____

_____

_____

_____

_____

_____

_____

_____

_____

_____

_____

_____

_____

_____

_____

_____

"Everything we hear is an opinion, not a fact. Everything we see is a perspective, not the truth."

—UNKNOWN

Often the serving sizes on food packages are determined arbitrarily, not based on how much a person should eat in one sitting. How do you decide how much food to eat? How would you like to determine how much is a serving for you?

_____

_____

_____

_____

_____

_____

_____

_____

_____

_____

_____

_____

_____

_____

_____

_____

_____

_____

Are there any foods or food groups that you do not allow yourself to eat at all? Are there any foods that you will not buy because you don't trust yourself around them? Where did these restrictions come from? Explore your thoughts and feelings about these foods.

_____

_____

_____

_____

_____

_____

_____

_____

_____

_____

_____

_____

_____

_____

_____

_____

_____

_____

MANTRA

We are not what we eat. We are vibrant, dynamic human beings who require nourishment for our bodies. We deserve to enjoy all foods.

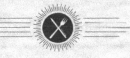

How do you feel after eating a food you consider "bad" or "unhealthy"? What thoughts arise? Do you have any thoughts that you need to behave or eat a certain way after eating this food? Where do these emotions and thoughts come from? Are they helpful or harmful?

_____

_____

_____

_____

_____

_____

_____

_____

_____

_____

_____

_____

_____

_____

_____

_____

_____

_____

_____

_____

What would it feel like to incorporate a food that you considered "forbidden" or "bad" on a regular basis?

_____

_____

_____

_____

_____

_____

_____

_____

_____

_____

_____

_____

_____

_____

_____

_____

_____

_____

_____

_____

Is there a food you would like to start incorporating? Detail a situation where you can envision eating this food when you can use the mindfulness techniques we've been practicing.

_____

_____

_____

_____

_____

_____

_____

_____

_____

_____

_____

_____

_____

_____

_____

_____

_____

_____

_____

_____

_____

PRACTICE

Take a deep breath and check in. Visualize yourself breaking a food rule. Notice your emotions and how they affect your body. Focus on your breathing, exhaling to release anxiety. What else can you do to release tension? Try stretching, placing your hand on your chest, and saying positive mantras. Remember not to believe every thought that arises. Respond to any negative thoughts with self-compassion.

What steps can you take to start dismantling old food rules that are no longer helping you? What rules can you start with? Include one action you can take today.

_____

_____

_____

_____

_____

_____

_____

_____

_____

_____

_____

_____

_____

_____

_____

_____

_____

_____

_____

"What you think of yourself is much more important than what others think of you."

—LUCIUS ANNAEUS SENECA

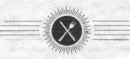

If negative thoughts or feelings come up after you break a food rule, how can you support yourself through this experience? Write three mantras or affirmations that you can repeat to yourself if negative thoughts or emotions arise.

_____

_____

_____

_____

_____

_____

_____

_____

_____

_____

_____

_____

_____

_____

_____

_____

_____

_____

_____

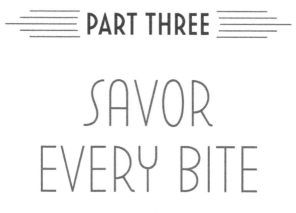

PART THREE

SAVOR EVERY BITE

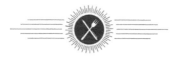

ating food is inherently pleasurable. Our brains are wired to reward us for eating because our bodies require nutrition to function. Think back to the infant who listens to their hunger and fullness cues without judgment. When the baby eats, not only does their discomfort from hunger dissipate, but feel-good chemicals also get released in their brain to reinforce the choice to cry out for food. Plus, the baby feels connection and comfort from their caregiver. Of course babies love to eat—it's an experience full of positive reinforcement! As adults, our brains release the same neurochemicals to positively reinforce eating. We also feel comforted by favorite foods and experience connection with loved ones during meals. However, dieting tells us that we are machines who only need to eat "perfectly" to achieve health. This distances us from the enjoyment we feel from eating delicious food. We don't eat only for biological reasons—we enjoy food because of the wonderful tastes, scents, textures, and temperatures we experience while eating. Different foods also elicit memories and emotions within us, reminding us of past experiences or loved ones, or help us feel connected with our culture of origin or places we have traveled. Our diet-obsessed society tells us that emotional eating is wrong, when in fact, food has provided us comfort, human connection, and gratification since we were infants. Sharing meals and dining out at restaurants are common ways we connect with others, celebrate holidays and special occasions, and share cultural traditions, but dieting tries to make us feel guilty about it. The truth is, we deserve to enjoy our food and all the flavors, sensations, nostalgia, and connections that come with it. This section focuses on staying present so we can find gratitude and rediscover enjoyment with meals.

"Wear gratitude like a cloak and it will feed every corner of your life."

—RUMI

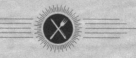

What are your favorite foods? Are any of your current favorite foods the same from your childhood? What emotions and memories arise when you eat your favorite foods?

_____

_____

_____

_____

_____

_____

_____

_____

_____

_____

_____

_____

_____

_____

_____

_____

_____

_____

_____

What foods do you eat regularly that make you feel satisfied? Consider whether the food makes you feel physically satisfied, if it satisfies a craving, or if it fits a favorite flavor profile or texture.

_____

_____

_____

_____

_____

_____

_____

_____

_____

_____

_____

_____

_____

_____

_____

_____

_____

_____

_____

In our busy lives, we can take our food for granted without appreciating where it comes from, the pleasure of its great taste, or how it nourishes our bodies. What do you love about food? How can you incorporate more food appreciation into your mindset?

_____

_____

_____

_____

_____

_____

_____

_____

_____

_____

_____

_____

_____

_____

_____

_____

_____

_____

PRACTICE

Choose a food that brings you joy when you eat it. Take time to check in with yourself. Consciously feel gratitude for this moment, your food, and your body. Then notice how the food looks and smells. Appreciate where this food comes from or how it was made. Chew your first bite slowly. Notice the food's flavor, texture, and temperature. Continue eating and see if the flavor and texture change over time. Notice any positive emotions or memories the food evokes. If negative or critical thoughts and feelings come into mind while eating, notice these associations and replace them with your intention of gratitude as you return your focus to your meal. Continue eating until you are satisfied, then check in with your physical sensations, thoughts, and emotions again. If negative emotions continue to come up, journal about where these emotions may be coming from.

Cravings sometimes happen for a reason. For instance, you may long for carbohydrates after a particularly protein-filled meal. It's also common to crave protein after physical activity when your body is building and repairing muscle. Explore how some of your food preferences or cravings might be meaningful for your health.

_____

_____

_____

_____

_____

_____

_____

_____

_____

_____

_____

_____

_____

_____

_____

_____

_____

Caring for our bodies' needs requires us to plan ahead. How can you plan meals and snacks that are satisfying? Consider what tastes you want at different times of the day, which foods keep you satisfied longer, and what foods you can take on the go or with limited time to prepare.

_____

_____

_____

_____

_____

_____

_____

_____

_____

_____

_____

_____

_____

_____

_____

_____

_____

_____

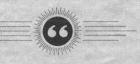

"It does not matter how slowly you go so long as you do not stop."

—CONFUCIUS

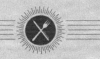

Let's explore our eating environments. Where do you typically eat your meals and snacks? Consider where you eat during the week and on the weekends. Include all details about the environments and your typical feelings, such as whether you are comfortable, distracted, stressed, alone, or with others.

_____

_____

_____

_____

_____

_____

_____

_____

_____

_____

_____

_____

_____

_____

_____

_____

_____

Considering the environments you detailed in the last entry, what improvements can you make? How can you make the dining experience more appealing and enjoyable? (Some ideas might include comfortable seating, removing distractions, eating with loved ones, or playing peaceful music.)

_____

_____

_____

_____

_____

_____

_____

_____

_____

_____

_____

_____

_____

_____

_____

_____

_____

_____

Which environments lend themselves to staying mindful? What can you do to eliminate distractions and allow yourself to check in and feel connected to your body throughout the meal?

_____

_____

_____

_____

_____

_____

_____

_____

_____

_____

_____

_____

_____

_____

_____

_____

_____

_____

_____

_____

MEDITATION

Is there a favorite food that you don't know how to incorporate mindfully? Consider how you can create an ideal environment to try the food without being overly hungry or full. Would you try it with a loved one? Do you want to try it at a restaurant or at home first? For example, let's use one of my favorite foods: chocolate. When deciding how to eat chocolate mindfully, start by getting a few types of chocolate that may be enjoyable. Allow yourself to take a bite or two of each chocolate and consider which types you like the most. Then, choose your favorite types and eat them slowly, taking note of how many chocolates it takes to be satisfied. Check in with yourself. What sensations and emotions are you feeling? Don't judge yourself for enjoying the chocolate (or whatever it may be) or for focusing on your favorites and not finishing the half-eaten food that was not as enjoyable. Allow yourself to break rules to learn how to eat the food in the most satisfying way.

A balanced plate means choosing foods that are satisfying to our bodies, our taste buds, and our emotions. We're not confined only to "healthy superfoods"; instead we can incorporate a variety of foods with carbohydrates, protein, and fat. How can you honor your choices about foods that satisfy you without judgment?

_____

_____

_____

_____

_____

_____

_____

_____

_____

_____

_____

_____

_____

_____

_____

_____

_____

Mindfulness, unlike dieting, isn't a mindset that requires per-
fection. Situations arise where we can't be mindful. What is a
situation you encountered recently where you didn't listen to
your hunger/fullness cues? What was that like for you?

_____

_____

_____

_____

_____

_____

_____

_____

_____

_____

_____

_____

_____

_____

_____

_____

_____

_____

_____

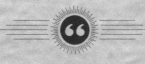

*"You are very powerful, provided
you know how powerful you are."*

—YOGI BHAJAN

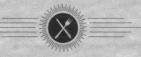

How can you be kind to yourself when you become uncomfortably hungry or uncomfortably full? Write some supportive mantras to reinforce that mindfulness is a process and there are no failures or missteps.

_____

_____

_____

_____

_____

_____

_____

_____

_____

_____

_____

_____

_____

_____

_____

_____

_____

_____

_____

All humans eat for emotional reasons, such as seeking comfort, enjoying social connection, celebrating cultural traditions, and feeling nostalgic. How do your positive emotions, such as happiness, gratitude, or celebration, influence your hunger and fullness cues? Do they affect what, when, or how much you eat?

_____

_____

_____

_____

_____

_____

_____

_____

_____

_____

_____

_____

_____

_____

_____

_____

_____

_____

_____

MANTRA

All food is nutritious, and breaks down into carbohydrates, protein, and fat. My body knows what to do with all the food it receives. I trust it.

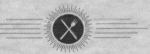

How do negative emotions affect what, when, or how much you eat? Consider stress, anxiety, boredom, sadness, and other feelings.

_____

_____

_____

_____

_____

_____

_____

_____

_____

_____

_____

_____

_____

_____

_____

_____

_____

_____

_____

_____

There are times when eating due to emotions may not be helpful. Can you think of a situation where you ate to cope with negative emotions? What emotions were coming up for you? How did food help? How did it not help?

_____

_____

_____

_____

_____

_____

_____

_____

_____

_____

_____

_____

_____

_____

_____

_____

_____

_____

_____

What are your coping mechanisms for negative emotions? How do you allow yourself to process and respect these emotions? (Coping mechanisms may include talking with a loved one, working with a therapist, taking necessary breaks, or writing in a journal.)

_____

_____

_____

_____

_____

_____

_____

_____

_____

_____

_____

_____

_____

_____

_____

_____

_____

_____

_____

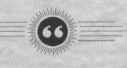

"Whatever you are doing, love yourself for doing it. Whatever you are feeling, love yourself for feeling it."

—THADDEUS GOLAS

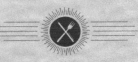

Are there situations where you would no longer like to rely on food for comfort? How can you be proactive in knowing when to use your coping techniques?

_____

_____

_____

_____

_____

_____

_____

_____

_____

_____

_____

_____

_____

_____

_____

_____

_____

_____

_____

PRACTICE

Write a thank-you letter to food. You can offer gratitude to all foods for providing you with nourishment or focus on a favorite food or food-related tradition that has been meaningful for you. If emotional eating resonates with you, the letter could thank food for how it has comforted you during difficult times.

What systems can you put into place to support you in having a positive, balanced relationship with food? For instance, how can you make mealtimes, grocery shopping, or food preparation more enjoyable? How can you incorporate more favorite foods and gratitude for your food?

_____

_____

_____

_____

_____

_____

_____

_____

_____

_____

_____

_____

_____

_____

_____

_____

_____

_____

_____

PART FOUR

A LIFETIME OF HEALTH AND HAPPINESS

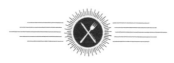

Our image-focused culture provides an ever-changing definition of what "perfect" eating looks like. It tells us that eating habits that are not "perfect" are wrong, and bodies that do not appear "perfect" are unhealthy. However, these unrealistic expectations cause us to diet and doubt our bodies' internal signals. Our brains and other organs constantly send one another messages so our bodies function optimally. For example, as we mindfully eat a meal, we become accustomed to the taste and our brains release fewer feel-good chemicals, so we experience less enjoyment as our bodies become satisfied.[9] Imagine feeling thirsty after being outside on a hot day. The first sip of cold water may taste like the best water you've ever had. As you continue drinking and your stomach fills with water, it may taste less amazing and more like plain water. If you have limited access to water, you may drink more water because you don't know when you'll be able to have more. The same happens with food! If you eat pasta for the first time after it's been forbidden due to a diet, it might taste like the best pasta you've ever eaten. Then, as you keep eating it, the pasta may start to lose its novelty if it's not actually a favorite dish. But if we are listening to our bodies' cues and know that pasta (and all foods) are always allowed, we can savor our food until we are satisfied (and have more whenever we want).

By adapting a mindful mentality emphasizing self-compassion, we learn how to take care of our bodies, minds, and emotions. We can deepen the connection we have with ourselves and our loved ones by remaining present and growing our empathy and gratitude. Shifting our mindset is difficult, requiring us to check in with ourselves continually and address the inner critic that comes up. In my life, transforming my inner voice from a bully to one of a friend has given me the strength to live in a way that feels meaningful and true to myself. This section will help you develop a sustainable mindfulness practice by building awareness of your inner voice, extending mindfulness to other parts of your life, and addressing challenges with self-compassion.

*"People who love to eat
are always the best people."*

—JULIA CHILD

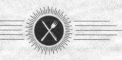

Reread your earliest entries in this journal. Are your thoughts about food different from when you started journaling? Discuss how your beliefs and feelings about food and mindfulness have changed.

_____

_____

_____

_____

_____

_____

_____

_____

_____

_____

_____

_____

_____

_____

_____

_____

_____

_____

_____

_____

Since starting this journal, what barriers have you encountered? How are you working on overcoming them?

_____

_____

_____

_____

_____

_____

_____

_____

_____

_____

_____

_____

_____

_____

_____

_____

_____

_____

_____

_____

_____

As we make significant shifts in our behavior, our critical voice can become louder and more intense. What emotions are coming up as you make changes? Are there any damaging food-related thoughts that you are struggling with? Write out any destructive thoughts related to food or self-image.

PRACTICE

Look at the damaging thoughts from the last prompt. Would you ever say these phrases to a beloved friend? Of course not! So why do we speak to ourselves this way? If your friend said this about themselves, what would you say to challenge it and encourage them to be kind to themselves? This is called reframing a thought. Review the thoughts from the previous prompt and reframe them as if you're talking to a friend.

How was the practice of thought reframing for you? What emotions came up? How can you apply this practice to change the way you talk to and think about yourself?

_____

_____

_____

_____

_____

_____

_____

_____

_____

_____

_____

_____

_____

_____

_____

_____

_____

_____

_____

_____

_____

_____

_____

What messages are you getting from the news, entertainment, or social media that are damaging to your self-image or food-related beliefs? How can you change what media you're receiving? (If you're stuck, there are some resources at the end of this journal to use as a starting point.)

_____

_____

_____

_____

_____

_____

_____

_____

_____

_____

_____

_____

_____

_____

_____

_____

_____

_____

_____

"*And how does one abide with one's heart imbued with loving-kindness extending outward in one direction? Just as one would feel friendliness on seeing a dearly beloved friend, so does one extend loving-kindness to all creatures.*"

—BUDDHA

Our thoughts reflect how we talk about ourselves and the world around us. How do you talk about food with your family, friends, and coworkers? How would you like your conversations about food to change?

_____

_____

_____

_____

_____

_____

_____

_____

_____

_____

_____

_____

_____

_____

_____

_____

_____

_____

_____

How can you share your mindfulness practice with others to deepen your connection with them? Are there certain loved ones you would like to start sharing with? How can you utilize them as a support system?

_____

_____

_____

_____

_____

_____

_____

_____

_____

_____

_____

_____

_____

_____

_____

_____

_____

_____

_____

_____

In our culture, people can be very opinionated about the "right" and "wrong" way to eat and can try to push what "works" for them onto others. However, no one knows what's best for your body except for you. How will you react if family, friends, and coworkers are resistant or skeptical when you discuss your mindfulness practice or a balanced attitude toward food? Write three responses you can use to assert your choices.

_____

_____

_____

_____

_____

_____

_____

_____

_____

_____

_____

_____

_____

_____

_____

_____

_____

_____

_____

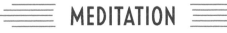

MEDITATION

Let's practice a brief, modern version of a Buddhist meditation called *metta bhavana*, or the cultivation of loving-kindness toward oneself and others. Sit comfortably, check in with yourself, and notice your breath. Visualize a loved one sitting with you—a person or animal who brings you comfort, calmness, and joy. See them next to you and send them love. Say the following out loud or in your mind: "I wish you safety and protection from fear and danger. I wish you health and well-being. I wish you great joy and peace." Now imagine your loved one sending this love back to you. Repeat these phrases, envisioning them sending you their well wishes. Now visualize yourself sending this love to all beings in the world. Repeat the phrases, imagining your well wishes touching everyone who needs this love and support.

How can you extend mindfulness to other parts of your life? Some examples include taking mindful walks with a loved one, starting a meditation practice, and doing yoga or another physical activity that is calming or enjoyable.

_____

_____

_____

_____

_____

_____

_____

_____

_____

_____

_____

_____

_____

_____

_____

_____

_____

_____

_____

What helps you feel present, connected, and safe in your body? What actions can you take to feel at one with your body and respectful of your needs at mealtimes or at times when you are experiencing negative emotions?

_____

_____

_____

_____

_____

_____

_____

_____

_____

_____

_____

_____

_____

_____

_____

_____

_____

_____

"Love yourself first, and everything else falls into line. You really have to love yourself to get anything done in this world."

—LUCILLE BALL

The idea of self-care means taking time for activities that bring us joy and help us feel our best physically, mentally, and emotionally. Some types of self-care are getting adequate sleep, going to medical or therapy appointments, making time for creative projects, getting a massage, or spending time with loved ones. What can you do for self-care? Describe at least three types of self-care you can do every week.

_____

_____

_____

_____

_____

_____

_____

_____

_____

_____

_____

_____

_____

_____

_____

_____

_____

_____

_____

Without doing any activities, how can you provide self-care within your own thoughts?

_____

_____

_____

_____

_____

_____

_____

_____

_____

_____

_____

_____

_____

_____

_____

_____

_____

_____

_____

_____

_____

Our critical inner voices tend to fixate on our appearances. Consider how much our bodies do for us. Our eyes allow us to see loved ones. Our lungs take in fresh air to oxygenate our blood, which our hearts pump throughout our bodies. Describe all the ways you appreciate your body. What steps can you take today to better care for and appreciate your body?

_____

_____

_____

_____

_____

_____

_____

_____

_____

_____

_____

_____

_____

_____

_____

_____

_____

_____

_____

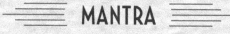

MANTRA

My body is amazing just as it is today. I deserve to take care of myself and my body.

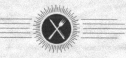

We often put off activities because we have been made to feel our bodies are inadequate and we feel self-conscious. What are you waiting to do until your body changes? What is in your way? What are your feelings around trying it now?

_____

_____

_____

_____

_____

_____

_____

_____

_____

_____

_____

_____

_____

_____

_____

_____

_____

If a beloved friend or child expressed the dreams and hesitations you expressed in the previous journal entry, how would you encourage them? Give yourself advice as if you were talking to a best friend.

_____

_____

_____

_____

_____

_____

_____

_____

_____

_____

_____

_____

_____

_____

_____

_____

_____

_____

"You yourself, as much as anybody in the entire universe, deserve your love and affection."

—BUDDHA

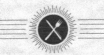

As much as we try to give ourselves time to eat mindfully, we will encounter periods of extreme stress. How are you going to continue to incorporate mindfulness even in times when you are busy or always on the go? Write five steps you can take to incorporate thoughts and actions of mindfulness and self-compassion that don't take substantial time and effort.

_____

_____

_____

_____

_____

_____

_____

_____

_____

_____

_____

_____

_____

_____

_____

_____

_____

_____

_____

PRACTICE

Write a love letter to yourself. Include what you like about yourself, what you are proud of, and how far you've come in overcoming obstacles in your life. Address your body and what it has done for you. Appreciate how much effort you've put into this journal and how far you've come.

Look back at your initial goals for this journal. What progress are you most proud of since starting this journal? What steps are you looking forward to taking next?

_____

_____

_____

_____

_____

_____

_____

_____

_____

_____

_____

_____

_____

_____

_____

_____

_____

_____

_____

_____

RESOURCES

Books:

Intuitive Eating by Elyse Resch, MS, RDN, and Evelyn Tribole, MS, RDN

The Intuitive Eating Workbook by Elyse Resch, MS, RDN, and Evelyn Tribole, MS, RDN

The Intuitive Eating Workbook for Teens by Elyse Resch, MS, RDN and Lucy Aphramor, PhD, RD

Body Respect by Linda Bacon, PhD and Lucy Aphramor, PhD, RD

Health at Every Size by Linda Bacon, PhD

Anti-Diet by Christy Harrison, MPH, RD

Body Kindness by Rebecca Scritchfield, RDN

The Gifts of Imperfection by Brene Brown, PhD, LMSW

The Mindful Self-Compassion Workbook by Kristin Neff, PhD, and Christopher Germer, PhD

Self-Compassion by Kristin Neff, PhD

Radical Acceptance by Tara Brach, PhD

Podcasts:

Love, Food hosted by Julie Duffy Dillon, RD

Food Psych hosted by Christy Harrison, MPH, RD

Dietitians Unplugged hosted by Aaron Flores, RDN, and Glenys Oyston, RDN

Body Kindness hosted by Rebecca Scritchfield, RDN

Unpacking Weight Science hosted by Fiona Willer, AdvAPD, AIDN

The Mindful Dietitian hosted by Fiona Sutherland, APD

The BodyLove Project hosted by Jessi Haggerty, RDN

Directories for Finding Providers Specializing in Disordered Eating:

Academy of Eating Disorders. aedweb.org.

Association for Size Diversity and Health. sizediversityandhealth.org.

International Association for Eating Disorder Professionals. iaedp.com.

International Federation of Eating Disorder Dietitians. eddietitians.com.

Intuitive Eating. intuitiveeating.org.

National Eating Disorders Association. nationaleatingdisorders.org.

Meditation Apps and Websites:

Aura. aurahealth.io.

Calm. calm.com.

Headspace. headspace.com.

Mindful. mindful.org.

UCLA Mindful. uclahealth.org/marc/mindful-meditations.

REFERENCES

1. Tribole, Evelyn, and Elyse Resch. *Intuitive Eating: A Revolutionary Program that Works*. New York, NY: St. Martin's Griffin, 1995.

2. Bacon, Linda, and Lucy Aphramor. "Weight Science: Evaluating the Evidence for a Paradigm Shift." *Nutrition Journal* 10, no. 9 (January 2011). www.nutritionj.com/content/10/1/9

3. Schaefer, Julie T., and Amy B. Magnuson. "A Review of Interventions that Promote Eating by Internal Cues." *Journal of the Academy of Nutrition and Dietetics* 114, no. 5 (May 2014): 734-760. doi:10.1016/j.jand.2013.12.024

4. Tylka, Tracy L., Rachel A. Annunziato, Deb Burgard, Sigrún Daníelsdóttir, Ellen Shuman, Chad Davis, and Rachel M. Calogero. "The Weight-Inclusive versus Weight-Normative Approach to Health: Evaluating the Evidence for Prioritizing Well-Being over Weight Loss." *Journal of Obesity* 2014 (July 2014). doi:10.1155/2014/983495

5. Jansen, Esther, Sandra Mulkens, Yvette Emond, and Anita Jansen. "From the Garden of Eden to the Land of Plenty: Restriction of Fruit and Sweets Intake Leads to Increased Fruit and Sweets Consumption in Children." *Appetite* 51, no. 3 (November 2008): 570-575. doi:10.1016/j.appet.2008.04.012

6. Keeler, Chelsey L., Richard D. Mattes, and Sze-Yen Tan. "Anticipatory and Reactive Responses to Chocolate Restriction in Frequent Chocolate Consumers." *Obesity* 23, no. 6 (May 2015): 1130-1135. doi:10.1002/oby.21098

7. Denny, Kara N., Katie Loth, Marla E. Eisenberg, and Dianne Neumark-Sztainer. "Intuitive Eating in Young Adults. Who is Doing it, and How is it Related to Disordered Eating Behaviors?" *Appetite* 60, no. 1 (January 2013): 13-9. doi:10.1016/j.appet.2012.09.029

8. Neumark-Sztainer, Dianne, Melanie Wall, Nicole I. Larson, Marla E. Eisenberg, and Katie Loth. "Dieting and Disordered Eating Behaviors from Adolescence to Young Adulthood: Findings from a 10-Year Longitudinal Study." *Journal of the American Dietetic Association* 111, no. 7 (July 2011): 1004-1011. doi:10.1016/j.jada.2011.04.012

9. Brunstrom, Jeffrey M., and Gemma L. Mitchell. "Effects of Distraction on the Development of Satiety." *British Journal of Nutrition* 96, no. 4 (October 2006): 761-769. doi:10.1079 /BJN20061880

GRATITUDE

T hank you to my parents for giving me life and supporting me in living it in my own way, even when I'm not sure what that is exactly. I love you. Thank you to my family for your support during the writing process and throughout my life. I love you all. I'd especially like to thank my husband, who somehow manifested this writing dream of mine into a reality. I love you, and I like you. Thank you to my dear friends who laugh with me, cry with me, and share your lives with me. I appreciate your support so much, and I love you.

Thank you to the anti-diet and eating disorder dietitians and therapists who have provided ideas, support, or (more often) both during my writing process and my career. I'd particularly like to thank the members of the Intuitive Eating and Eating Disorder Registered Dietician supervision groups I attend and the group leaders, Elyse and Lauren. Thank you all for the amazing guidance, support, and inspiration in my career and in the topics discussed in this journal.

I'd also like to thank the experts in mindfulness, body respect, and the anti-diet movement who authored the books I've included as resources. You all walked fearlessly and blazed trails so that I could run down them in my work as a dietitian and in writing this journal.

Thank you to my editor, Lia, for your guidance and feedback as we made this journal a reality. Thank you to Elizabeth and the rest of the Callisto team for this opportunity and for your support.

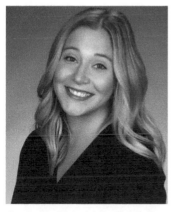

Alyssa Snow Callahan, MS, RDN, is a registered dietitian nutritionist and certified intuitive eating counselor specializing in eating disorders, mindful eating, and body image. She graduated with her master's degree in nutritional science from California State University at Los Angeles. She began her career as a dietitian working in inpatient and intensive care at Cedars-Sinai Medical Center in Los Angeles. She currently works for an eating disorder treatment center and has a private practice in Westlake Village, California. Alyssa is a member of the International Association of Eating Disorder Professionals, the International Federation of Eating Disorder Dietitians, and supervision groups for *Intuitive Eating* and eating disorder dietitians.

Originally from New Hampshire, Alyssa graduated from Boston University with a degree in communication and worked in health policy public affairs in Washington, D.C. before becoming a dietitian.

Alyssa enjoys yoga, eating Mexican food with her family, traveling with her husband, Brendan, laughing with her friends, and napping with her dogs, Ellie and Joy, and her cats Meru and Jongo.

You can visit Alyssa's website at **alyssacallahanrd.com** or follow her on Instagram at @EDrecoveryRD.

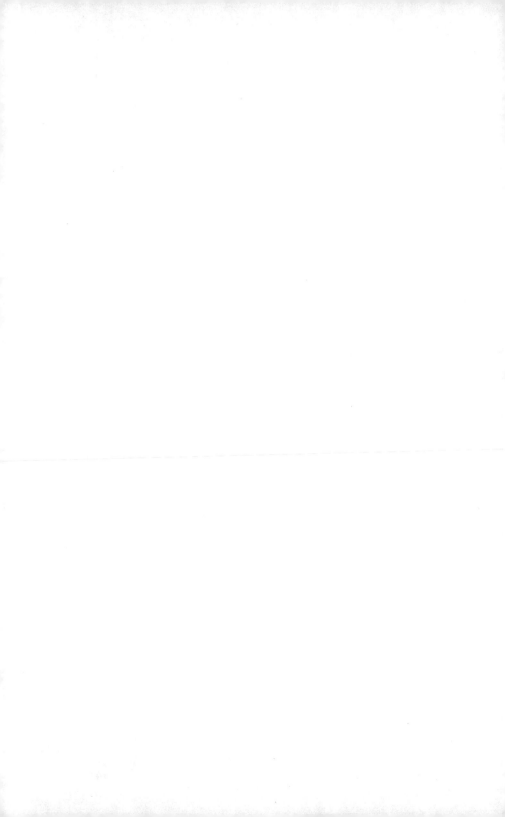